# GOODBEY, FERTILITY BOOSTER!:

## "Taking Control of Menopause via Diet, Hormones, and Inner Voice"

Hope Sylvan

extended by sales representatives or written sales materials. The advice and strategies contained herein may not be suitable for your situation. You should consult with a professional when appropriate. Neither the publisher nor the author shall be liable for any loss of profit or any other commercial damages, including but not limited to special, incidental, consequential, personal, or other damages.

# TABLE OF CONTENT

# TABLE OF CONTENT

Chapter 10:
Embracing the Journey
Celebrating Personal Growth
Finding Joy in Midlife
Inspiring Stories of Women Thriving in Menopause

Conclusion.

# Introduction

Welcome to " Goodbye, Fertility Booster!: "Taking Control of Menopause via Diet, Hormones, and Inner Voice"
 Hope Sylvan. In this introductory section, we delve into the author's unique perspective on menopause, setting the stage for a comprehensive exploration of this transformative phase in a woman's life.

# Author's Perspective on Menopause

Hope Sylvan, a seasoned expert in holistic health, shares her insightful perspective on menopause, drawing from years of experience and a deep understanding of women's wellness. Through her lens, menopause is not merely a collection of symptoms but a powerful transition—one that can be navigated with grace and vitality. Sylvan's approach emphasizes embracing this natural evolution, empowering women to thrive through informed choices and holistic well-being.

# The Importance of Nutrition, Hormones, and Self-Advocacy

In this book, nutrition takes center stage as a crucial element in managing menopausal symptoms. Sylvan explores the impact of dietary choices on hormonal balance and provides practical insights into crafting meal plans that support overall health during this life stage. Furthermore, the discussion extends to the realm of hormones, examining both traditional and natural approaches to maintaining equilibrium.

A core theme throughout this book is self-advocacy. Sylvan underscores the significance of women actively participating in their health journey, advocating for their well-being, and making informed decisions. This involves open communication with healthcare professionals, understanding treatment options, and embracing a proactive role in achieving optimal health throughout menopause.

As we embark on this journey through menopause, Hope Sylvan invites you to consider a holistic and empowering perspective—one that embraces nutrition, hormones, and self-advocacy as essential tools in mastering this transformative phase. Get ready to navigate menopause with confidence, vitality, and a renewed sense of well-being.

# Chapter 1

# Understanding Menopause

## Definition and Phases of Menopause

Menopause, a natural biological transition in women's lives, marks the end of their reproductive years. It is characterized by a gradual decline in the production of ovarian hormones, primarily estrogen and progesterone. This hormonal shift leads to a range of physical and emotional changes.

The menopausal transition typically occurs between the ages of 45 and 55, with the average age being 51. The process can take several years, encompassing three distinct phases:

**Premenopause:** This phase begins several years before menopause and is characterized by fluctuating hormone levels and irregular periods.

**Perimenopause:** The perimenopausal phase, typically lasting 4-8 years, is the transitional period leading up to menopause. During this phase, estrogen levels decline significantly, leading to various symptoms.

**Postmenopause:** Postmenopause is defined as the period following one year without menstruation. During this phase, estrogen levels stabilize, and symptoms may gradually subside.

# Common Symptoms and Challenges

The hormonal changes associated with menopause can manifest in a variety of symptoms, including:

**Hot flashes:** Sudden, intense sensations of heat, often accompanied by sweating, flushing, and rapid heartbeat.

**Night sweats:** Hot flashes that occur during sleep, disrupt sleep patterns, and cause discomfort.

**Vaginal dryness:** Reduced estrogen levels can lead to thinning and dryness of vaginal tissues, causing discomfort during intercourse.

**Mood swings:** Hormonal fluctuations can contribute to emotional instability, irritability, and mood swings.

**Sleep disturbances:** Sleep problems, such as insomnia, are common during menopause due to hot flashes, night sweats, and anxiety.

**Changes in libido:** Reduced estrogen levels can lead to a decline in sexual desire and arousal.

**Cognitive changes:** Some women may experience mild memory lapses, difficulty concentrating, or foggy thinking.

**Osteoporosis:** The decline in estrogen can increase the risk of osteoporosis, a condition characterized by weak and brittle bones.

These symptoms can vary in intensity and duration among women, making menopause a unique and personal experience.

# Embracing Menopause as a New Chapter

Menopause is not a disease or an ending but rather a natural transition in women's lives. It marks the end of one chapter and the beginning of another, offering an opportunity for personal growth, self-discovery, and new experiences.

By understanding the changes that occur during menopause and developing strategies to manage symptoms, women can navigate this transition with confidence and embrace the opportunities it presents.

# Chapter 2

# Nutrition for Menopause

## Impact of Diet on Menopausal Symptoms

Nutrition plays a crucial role in managing menopausal symptoms and promoting overall well-being during this transitional phase of life. A balanced and nutrient-rich diet can help alleviate symptoms, improve energy levels, and support long-term health.

**Hormonal Balance:** Certain dietary components can influence hormonal balance, reducing the severity of symptoms like hot flashes, mood swings, and sleep disturbances.

**Weight Management:** Maintaining a healthy weight can help reduce the risk of weight gain, a common concern during menopause.

**Bone Health:** Adequate intake of calcium, vitamin D, and other bone-building nutrients is essential to prevent osteoporosis, a condition that increases in risk after menopause.

**Overall Health:** A healthy diet contributes to overall well-being, reducing the risk of chronic diseases like heart disease, stroke, and type 2 diabetes, which become more prevalent with age.

# Superfoods for Hormonal Balance

Incorporating certain nutrient-rich foods into your diet can support hormonal balance and alleviate menopausal symptoms:

**Flaxseeds and Soy Products:** These foods contain phytoestrogens, plant compounds that mimic the effects of estrogen, potentially helping to reduce hot flashes and other symptoms.

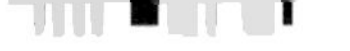

**Fatty Fish:** Salmon, sardines, and mackerel are rich sources of omega-3 fatty acids, which have anti-inflammatory properties and may help improve mood and reduce hot flashes.

**Cruciferous Vegetables:** Broccoli, Brussels sprouts, and kale contain indole-3-carbinol, a compound that may help regulate estrogen metabolism.

**Legumes:** Beans, lentils, and peas provide protein, fiber, and vitamins, supporting overall health and potentially alleviating menopausal symptoms.

**Berries:** These fruits are rich in antioxidants, which can help protect against cell damage and reduce inflammation.

# Meal Plans and Recipes for Menopausal Health

Here's a sample meal plan incorporating nutrient-rich foods that support menopausal health:

**Breakfast:**

Oatmeal with berries and flaxseeds

**Lunch:**

Salad with grilled salmon and quinoa

**Dinner:**

Roasted chicken breast with steamed vegetables and brown rice

**Snacks:**

Nuts and seeds
Fruits and vegetables
Yogurt with fruit and granola

These recipes provide a starting point for creating a customized meal plan tailored to individual preferences and dietary needs. Consult a healthcare professional or registered dietitian for personalized guidance.

# Chapter 3

# Hormones and Menopause

## Hormonal Changes During Menopause

Menopause is characterized by a decline in the production of ovarian hormones, primarily estrogen and progesterone. These hormonal changes lead to a range of physical and emotional symptoms.

**Hormone:** Estrogen

**Function:** Responsible for many of the secondary sex characteristics in women, including breast development, menstrual cycles, and bone health.

**Changes During Menopause:** Levels decline significantly.

**Symptoms:** Hot flas
hes, vaginal dryness, mood swings

**Hormone:** Progesterone

**Function:** Works in conjunction with estrogen to regulate the menstrual cycle and prepare the uterus for pregnancy.

**Changes During Menopause:** Levels also decline.

**Symptoms:** Irregular periods, other symptoms |

# Hormone Replacement Therapy (HRT)

Hormone replacement therapy (HRT) is a medical treatment that involves taking hormones to replace those that are naturally declining during menopause. HRT can be an effective way to manage menopausal symptoms, but it is important to discuss the risks and benefits with a healthcare professional.

# Types of HRT

There are two main types of HRT:

**Estrogen-only therapy:** This type of HRT is used for women who have had a hysterectomy, a surgical procedure that removes the uterus.

**Estrogen-progestin therapy:** This type of HRT is used for women who have not had a hysterectomy. Progestin is added to estrogen therapy to reduce the risk of endometrial cancer.

# Natural Approaches to Hormonal Balance

In addition to HRT, several natural approaches may help to balance hormones and alleviate menopausal symptoms. These include:

**Diet:** Eating a healthy diet that is rich in fruits, vegetables, whole grains, and lean protein can help to support overall health and well-being.

**Exercise:** Regular exercise can help to improve mood, reduce stress, and promote bone health.

**Stress management:** Finding healthy ways to manage stress, such as yoga, meditation, or spending time in nature, can help to reduce the severity of menopausal symptoms.

**Supplements:** Some supplements, such as vitamin D, calcium, and magnesium, may help to alleviate specific menopausal symptoms.

It is important to talk to a healthcare professional before taking any supplements, as some may interact with medications or have other side effects.

By understanding the hormonal changes that occur during menopause and exploring both conventional and natural approaches to managing symptoms, women can navigate this transition with confidence and maintain their overall well-being.

# Chapter 4

# Self-Advocacy in Menopause

## Communicating with Healthcare Professionals

Effective communication with healthcare professionals is crucial for navigating menopause and receiving optimal care. Here are some tips for fostering open and effective communication:

**Be Prepared:** Gather information about your symptoms, including when they started, how they affect your daily life, and any triggers you've noticed.

**Ask Questions:** Don't hesitate to ask questions, no matter how simple they may seem. Clarify any information you don't understand and seek explanations for treatment options.

**Express Concerns:** Openly share your concerns about menopausal symptoms, their impact on your quality of life, and any potential side effects of treatment options.

**Be Assertive:** Communicate your preferences regarding treatment approaches and involve yourself in decision-making.

**Seek Second Opinions:** If you have doubts or concerns about your current treatment plan, consider seeking a second opinion from another healthcare professional.

# Making Informed Decisions about Treatment

Informed decision-making is essential for managing menopause effectively. Here are some steps to making informed treatment decisions:

**Gather Information:** Educate yourself about menopause, treatment options, and their potential risks and benefits. Utilize reliable sources, such as medical journals, patient education websites, and reputable books.

**Discuss Options with Healthcare Providers:** Engage in open discussions with your healthcare providers about various treatment options, their suitability for your specific needs, and potential side effects.

**Consider Lifestyle Changes:** Explore lifestyle modifications, such as diet, exercise, and stress management techniques, as potential complementary or alternative approaches to manage symptoms.

**Weigh Risks and Benefits:** Carefully evaluate the potential risks and benefits of each treatment option in light of your individual circumstances, preferences, and health goals.

**Seek Support:** Consult with trusted friends, family members, or support groups for guidance and emotional support during the decision-making process.

### Advocating for Your Well-being

Self-advocacy is paramount in ensuring your well-being throughout menopause. Here are strategies to effectively advocate for yourself:

**Be Proactive:** Take charge of your healthcare by scheduling regular checkups, tracking your symptoms, and proactively communicating concerns to your healthcare providers.

**Set Goals:** Establish clear and measurable goals for managing your symptoms and improving your overall health and well-being.

**Empower Yourself:** Educate yourself about menopause, treatment options, and your rights as a patient to make informed decisions.

**Communicate Assertively:** Clearly express your preferences, concerns, and expectations to your healthcare providers.

**Don't Hesitate to Seek Clarification:** If you have doubts or questions, don't hesitate to ask for clarification or seek additional information from your healthcare providers.

**Seek Additional Support:** Consider seeking support from patient advocacy groups, online forums, or

counseling services to navigate menopause with confidence.

By cultivating effective communication with healthcare professionals, making informed treatment decisions, and advocating for their well-being, women can empower themselves to manage menopause effectively and maintain optimal health and well-being throughout this transition.

# Chapter 5

# Exercise and Menopause

## Importance of Physical Activity

Regular physical activity is an essential component of overall health and well-being, especially during menopause. Engaging in regular exercise offers a multitude of benefits for menopausal women, including:

**Improved Cardiovascular Health:** Exercise strengthens the heart and improves circulation, reducing the risk of heart disease, stroke, and high blood pressure.

**Weight Management:** Exercise helps maintain a healthy weight, which can alleviate menopausal symptoms and reduce the risk of chronic diseases associated with menopause.

**Stronger Bones and Muscles:** Exercise promotes bone density and muscle strength, reducing the risk of osteoporosis and sarcopenia, a condition characterized by muscle loss.

**Enhanced Mood and Reduced Stress:** Exercise releases endorphins, natural mood-boosting chemicals, and helps manage stress, which can alleviate menopausal symptoms like anxiety and mood swings.

**Improved Sleep Quality:** Regular exercise can promote better sleep patterns, which can be disrupted by menopausal symptoms like hot flashes and night sweats.

# Customizing Exercise Routines for Menopausal Women

When creating an exercise routine, it is crucial to consider individual preferences, fitness levels, and any underlying health conditions. Here are some tips for customizing exercise routines for menopausal women:

**Start Gradually:** Begin with low-impact exercises and gradually increase the intensity and duration of workouts as fitness improves.

**Variety is Key:** Incorporate a variety of exercises into your routine, including aerobic activities, strength training, and flexibility exercises.

**Find Enjoyable Activities:** Choose activities you find enjoyable and sustainable to maintain motivation and adherence to your exercise routine.

**Listen to Your Body:** Pay attention to your body's signals and rest when needed. Don't push yourself beyond your limits.

**Seek Professional Guidance:** Consult a healthcare professional or a certified personal trainer to develop an exercise plan tailored to your specific needs and goals.

# Yoga, Pilates, and Other Beneficial Practices

Specific exercise modalities can be particularly beneficial for menopausal women:

**Yoga:** Yoga combines physical postures, breathing techniques, and meditation, promoting flexibility, strength, balance, and stress reduction.

**Pilates:** Pilates focuses on strengthening the core muscles, improving posture, and enhancing overall body control.

**Tai Chi:** Tai Chi is a gentle, low-impact exercise that promotes balance, coordination, and stress reduction.

**Walking:** Walking is a simple yet effective form of exercise that can be done almost anywhere and at any time.

**Swimming:** Swimming is a low-impact exercise that is easy on the joints and provides a full-body workout.

**Dancing:** Dancing is a fun and enjoyable way to get exercise and improve cardiovascular health.

Incorporating these exercise modalities into your routine can effectively manage menopausal symptoms, promote overall health, and enhance your quality of life. Remember to consult with your healthcare provider before starting any new exercise program.

# Chapter 6

# Mind-Body Connection

## Managing Stress During Menopause

The hormonal fluctuations associated with menopause can contribute to increased stress levels, leading to anxiety, mood swings, and difficulty sleeping. Managing stress effectively is crucial for maintaining overall well-being during this transitional phase.

# Stress-Management Strategies

Here are some effective strategies for managing stress during menopause:

**Identify Stressors:** Recognize the situations, people, or thoughts that trigger stress in your life.

**Practice Relaxation Techniques:** Engage in relaxation techniques such as deep breathing, progressive muscle relaxation, or meditation to calm the mind and body.

**Prioritize Sleep:** Aim for 7-8 hours of quality sleep each night to promote relaxation and stress resilience.

**Engage in Regular Exercise:** Regular physical activity releases endorphins, natural mood boosters, and helps reduce stress levels.

**Nourish Your Body:** Eat a balanced diet rich in fruits, vegetables, and whole grains to provide your body with the nutrients it needs to cope with stress.

**Connect with Loved Ones:** Maintain strong social connections with family, friends, or support groups to provide emotional support and reduce feelings of isolation.

# Meditation and Mindfulness Practices

Meditation and mindfulness practices can be particularly effective in managing stress and enhancing emotional well-being during menopause.

**Meditation:** Meditation involves focusing your attention on the present moment, training your mind to resist distractions and cultivate inner peace.

**Mindfulness:** Mindfulness involves paying attention to your thoughts, feelings, and sensations without judgment, promoting self-awareness and acceptance.

### Mindfulness-Based Stress Reduction (MBSR):

MBSR is an eight-week program that combines meditation, mindfulness practices, and body awareness techniques to effectively manage stress.

## Cultivating Emotional Resilience

Emotional resilience is the ability to cope with and adapt to difficult emotions and life challenges. Strengthening emotional resilience can enhance your ability to navigate menopausal symptoms and maintain well-being.

**Practice Self-Compassion:** Be kind and understanding towards yourself, accepting that emotional ups and downs are a normal part of menopause.

**Challenge Negative Thoughts:** Identify and challenge negative thought patterns that contribute to stress and anxiety.

**Develop Coping Mechanisms:** Find healthy coping mechanisms, such as journaling, creative pursuits, or spending time in nature, to manage difficult emotions.

**Seek Professional Support:** If stress is significantly impacting your daily life, consider seeking professional support from a therapist or counselor.

By incorporating stress-management strategies, mindfulness practices, and emotional resilience techniques into your daily life, you can effectively manage stress, enhance emotional well-being, and navigate menopause with greater ease and confidence.

# Chapter 7

# Sleep Strategies for Menopause

## Understanding Sleep Disruptions

Sleep disturbances are a common symptom of menopause, affecting up to 60% of women during this transition. The hormonal changes associated with menopause, particularly the decline in estrogen levels, can disrupt sleep patterns and make it difficult to fall asleep, stay asleep, or get enough quality sleep.

# Common Sleep Disruptions During Menopause

**Symptom:** Hot flashes

**Description:** Sudden sensations of intense heat that can occur during sleep, causing night sweats and disrupting sleep patterns.

**Symptom:** Night sweats

**Description:** Excessive sweating that occurs during sleep, leading to discomfort and sleep disturbances.

**Symptom:** Anxiety and mood swings

**Description:** Anxiety and mood swings associated with menopause can make it difficult to relax and fall asleep.

**Symptom:** Changes in sleep patterns

**Description:** Sleep patterns may change during menopause, with some women experiencing insomnia (difficulty falling asleep) and others experiencing early morning awakenings.

# Creating a Sleep-Inducing Environment

Establishing a sleep-conducive environment can significantly improve sleep quality during menopause:

**Tip:** Maintain a regular sleep schedule

**Description:** Go to bed and wake up at the same time each day, even on weekends.

**Tip:** Establish a relaxing bedtime routine

**Description:** This may include taking a warm bath, reading a book, or listening to calming music.

**Tip:** Optimize sleep environment

**Description:** Create a dark, quiet, and cool bedroom. Use blackout curtains, earplugs, or a white noise machine if necessary.

**Tip:** Avoid caffeine and alcohol before bed

**Description:** These substances can interfere with sleep.

**Tip:** Engage in regular exercise

**Description:** Avoid strenuous activity close to bedtime.

**Tip:** Maintain a healthy diet

**Description:** Avoid heavy meals or sugary snacks close to bedtime.

# Natural Remedies for Better Sleep

In addition to creating a sleep-conducive environment, certain natural remedies may help improve sleep quality during menopause:

**Remedy:** Relaxation techniques

**Description:** Practice relaxation techniques such as deep breathing, progressive muscle relaxation, or meditation to promote relaxation and reduce stress before bed.

**Remedy:** Herbal remedies

**Description:** Consider herbal remedies such as chamomile tea or valerian root, which may have mild sedative effects.

**Remedy:** Melatonin

**Description:** Melatonin is a hormone that regulates sleep-wake cycles. Melatonin supplements may help regulate sleep patterns during menopause.

## Consulting a Healthcare Professional

If sleep disturbances persist despite implementing these strategies, consult a healthcare professional to rule out any underlying medical conditions and discuss additional treatment options.

By understanding the causes of sleep disruptions during menopause and implementing effective sleep strategies, women can improve their sleep quality and enhance their overall well-being during this transition.

# Chapter 8

# Sexual Health in Menopause

As women navigate the transformative landscape of menopause, Chapter 8 delves into a critical aspect often surrounded by silence and uncertainty—sexual health. Hope Sylvan carefully addresses the intricacies of this topic, offering insights, guidance, and practical solutions for embracing a fulfilling and satisfying intimate life during and after menopause.

# Addressing Changes in Libido

Menopause can usher in changes in libido, impacting one's desire and interest in sexual activities. Blum explores the physiological and hormonal shifts contributing to these changes, fostering an understanding that empowers women to navigate this aspect of their well-being with knowledge and confidence. Through candid discussions and expert advice, this section aims to dismantle taboos and encourage open conversations about libido shifts during menopause.

# Communication with Partners

Effective communication is paramount in maintaining healthy relationships, especially during the complex journey of menopause. This chapter guides readers through strategies for fostering open and honest communication with partners. Blum provides insights into expressing needs, navigating emotional aspects, and ensuring that both individuals feel supported and

understood as they navigate the changes in sexual dynamics that can accompany menopause.

# Solutions for Maintaining Intimacy

Arming women with practical tools, this section offers a spectrum of solutions for maintaining intimacy throughout menopause. From exploring different forms of intimacy to considering lifestyle adjustments, Blum provides a holistic approach to rekindling and sustaining the connection with one's partner. Whether through lifestyle changes, mindfulness practices, or seeking professional guidance, this chapter aims to empower women to proactively engage in and enjoy a healthy vibrant intimate life beyond menopause.

Chapter 8 invites readers to confront the challenges and possibilities surrounding sexual health during menopause, fostering a sense of empowerment, understanding, and connection. By addressing changes in libido, facilitating communication with partners, and offering practical solutions, this chapter contributes to a comprehensive guide for mastering menopause with confidence and vitality

# Chapter 9

# Navigating Work and Menopause

## Balancing Career Responsibilities

Menopause can bring about a myriad of physical and emotional changes, making it challenging to maintain a healthy work-life balance. However, with the right strategies and support, women can continue to thrive in their careers during this transition.

## Prioritize Self-Care:

**Schedule regular breaks:** Take short breaks throughout the day to step away from your desk, stretch, and clear your head.

**Engage in physical activity:** Regular exercise can help alleviate stress, improve sleep, and boost energy levels.

**Maintain a healthy diet:** Eating nutritious foods provides your body with the essential nutrients it needs to function optimally.

**Practice relaxation techniques:** Incorporate stress-management practices like mindfulness meditation or deep breathing into your daily routine.

## Effective Time Management:

**Plan and prioritize tasks:** Create a daily or weekly schedule to organize your workload and prioritize important tasks.

**Delegate responsibilities:** If possible, delegate tasks to colleagues or subordinates to free up your time for more critical responsibilities.

**Set realistic expectations:** Don't overload yourself; set achievable goals and avoid overcommitting.

**Utilize technology:** Take advantage of productivity tools and time-saving apps to streamline your workflow.

# Communicating with Employers and Colleagues

Open and honest communication with your employer and colleagues can help create a supportive work environment and reduce any stigma associated with menopause.

**Educate your employer**: Provide your employer with information about menopause and its potential impact on your work.

**Discuss workplace accommodations:** If necessary, discuss potential workplace accommodations, such as flexible work arrangements or access to private spaces.

**Seek support from colleagues:** Connect with colleagues who may be experiencing similar challenges or seek mentorship from experienced women.

# Strategies for Professional Success during Menopause

Despite the challenges, menopause can also be a time of personal and professional growth.

**Embrace your experience:** Use your accumulated knowledge and skills to mentor and guide others.

**Network and build relationships:** Expand your professional network and build strong relationships with colleagues and clients.

**Reassess your career goals:** Reflect on your long-term career aspirations and make adjustments as needed.

**Seek professional development opportunities:** Continuous learning can enhance your skills and boost your career prospects.

Remember, you are not alone. Many women successfully navigate menopause while maintaining fulfilling careers. With self-awareness, effective communication, and supportive strategies, you can continue to thrive professionally during this transition.

# Chapter 10

## Embracing the Journey

## Celebrating Personal Growth

Menopause marks a significant transition in a woman's life, often accompanied by a period of personal reflection and growth. As women navigate this change, they often gain a deeper understanding of themselves, their values, and their priorities.

**Emerging Strength and Resilience:** Many women experience a newfound sense of strength and resilience during menopause. They learn to adapt to change, manage stress effectively, and advocate for their needs.

**Enhanced Self-Awareness:** Menopause can prompt women to delve deeper into their self-awareness, developing a clearer understanding of their strengths, passions, and life aspirations.

**Embracing Authenticity:** Women often embrace their authentic selves during menopause, shedding societal expectations and embracing their individuality.

**Prioritizing Well-being:** Menopause can be a catalyst for prioritizing well-being, leading to healthier habits, stronger self-care practices, and a renewed appreciation for life's simple pleasures.

# Finding Joy in Midlife

Menopause doesn't signal the end of one's life; instead, it can usher in a period of renewed joy, fulfillment, and self-discovery.

**Rekindling Passions:** Women often rediscover passions and interests that may have been put on hold during their earlier years, pursuing hobbies, creative endeavors, and personal projects with renewed enthusiasm.

**Strengthening Relationships:** Menopause can provide an opportunity to strengthen relationships with loved ones, fostering deeper connections with family and friends.

**Embracing New Adventures:** Women may embark on new adventures, traveling, pursuing education, or starting new ventures, embracing the possibilities that midlife presents.

**Giving Back to Others:** Many women find fulfillment in giving back to their communities, volunteering their time, sharing their knowledge, and making a positive impact on the world around them.

# Inspiring Stories of Women Thriving in Menopause

Countless women have transformed their experiences during menopause into stories of resilience, growth, and inspiration. Their journeys serve as a testament to the strength and adaptability of women during this transition.

**Oprah Winfrey:** Media mogul, philanthropist, and global icon Oprah Winfrey has openly shared her experiences with menopause, advocating for open dialogue and dispelling misconceptions.

**Emma Watson:** Actress and activist Emma Watson has championed women's health and well-being, advocating for menopause education and support.

**Michelle Obama:** Former First Lady Michelle Obama has spoken about the importance of self-care and embracing change during menopause.

**Susan Sarandon:** Actress Susan Sarandon has challenged age stereotypes and embraced her authentic self throughout her life, including during menopause.

**Jane Fonda:** Actress, activist, and fitness icon Jane Fonda has promoted healthy aging and self-acceptance, encouraging women to embrace their bodies and lives at any age.

These women, along with countless others, exemplify the power of resilience, self-acceptance, and embracing the journey of menopause. Their stories inspire women to navigate this transition with confidence, grace, and a renewed appreciation for life's possibilities.

# Conclusion

## Reflections on the Menopausal Journey

Menopause, a natural transition in a woman's life, marks the end of her reproductive years and the beginning of a new chapter. While it can be accompanied by physical and emotional challenges, it also presents an opportunity for personal growth, self-discovery, and embracing new possibilities.

**A Time of Transformation:** Menopause is not an ending but a transformation, a time to shed societal expectations and embrace authenticity. It's a chance to

redefine priorities, pursue passions, and rediscover oneself.

**A Journey of Resilience:** Navigating menopause requires resilience, adaptability, and self-compassion. It's about finding strength in the face of change, seeking support when needed, and celebrating victories along the way.

**A Celebration of Wisdom and Experience:** Menopause brings with it a wealth of wisdom, experience, and self-awareness. It's a time to honor the contributions of women and their enduring impact on society.

# Encouragement for Women Navigating Menopause

To the women embarking on or currently navigating the menopausal journey, remember that you are not alone. Countless women have walked this path before you, and many are walking beside you now. Embrace this transition with courage, grace, and a sense of adventure.

**Embrace Your Strengths:** Recognize your inner strength and resilience, the qualities that have carried

you through life's challenges. Honor your accomplishments and the wisdom you have gained.

**Seek Support and Connection:** Surround yourself with supportive friends, family, and healthcare professionals. Connect with other women experiencing menopause, sharing experiences and offering mutual encouragement.

**Prioritize Well-being:** Nurture your physical and emotional well-being. Engage in regular exercise, maintain a healthy diet, practice stress-management techniques, and prioritize quality sleep.

**Celebrate Your Authentic Self:** Embrace your individuality and authentic self, shedding societal expectations and embracing your true essence.

**Embrace the Possibilities:** Menopause is not an end but a beginning, a time to explore new possibilities, pursue passions, and redefine your life's journey.

Remember, you are not defined by your hormones or your age. You are a woman of strength, resilience, and wisdom, capable of embracing change, navigating challenges, and thriving in every chapter of your life.